Dump Dinners

101 Easy, Delicious, and Healthy Meals Put Together in 30 Minutes or Less!

RUTH FERGUSON

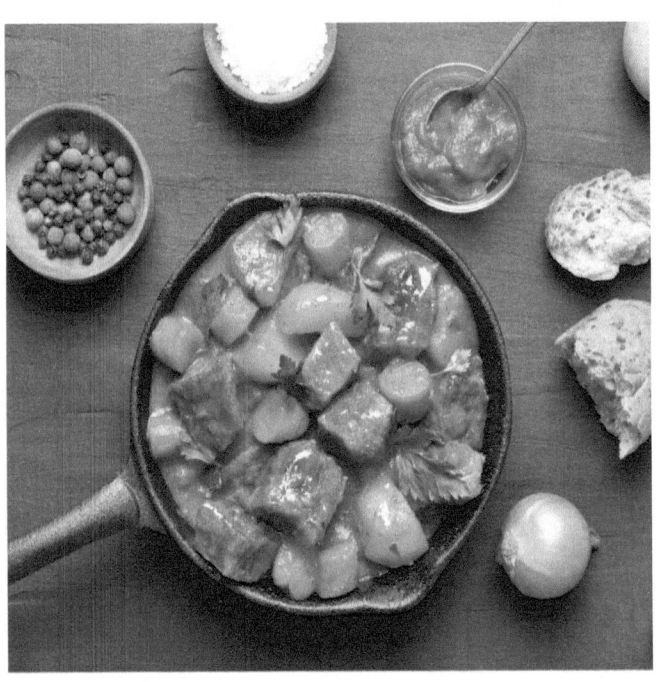

Copyright © 2014 Paradise Books

All rights reserved.

In no way is it legal to reproduce, duplicate or transmit any part of this document in either electronic means or in printed format. Recording of this publication is strictly prohibited and any storage of this document is not allowed unless with written permission from the publisher. All rights reserved.

The information provided herein is stated to be truthful and consistent, in that any liability, in terms of inattention or otherwise, by any usage or abuse of any policies, processes or directions contained within is the solitary and utter responsibility of the recipient reader. Under no circumstances will any legal responsibility or blame be held against the publisher for any reparation, damages or monetary loss due to the information herein, either directly or indirectly.

Respective authors own all copyrights not held by the publisher.

The information herein is offered for informational purposes solely and is universal as so. The presentation of the information is without contract or any type of guarantee assurance.

The trademarks that are used are without any consent and the publication of the trademark is without permission or backing by the trademark owner. All trademarks and brands within this book are for clarifying purposes only and are owned by the owners themselves, not affiliated with this document.

CONTENTS

Introduction		i
Chapter 1	What's For Dinner?	1
Chapter 2	Chicken Dinners	5
	Creamy Chicken Casserole	5
	Italian Chicken and Rice	7
	Mexican Chicken Lasagna	8
	Creamy Peanut Chicken	9
	Chicken Mushroom Casserole	10
	Spicy Lime Chicken	11
	Easiest Chicken Casserole	12
	Chicken, Tomato, and Rice Casserole	13
	Honey Onion Ginger Chicken	14
	Monterey Jack Chicken and Rice Casserole	15
	All-in-One Chicken Dinner	16
	General Tsao's Chicken	17
	Chicken and Stuffing	18
	Apricot Chicken	19
	Amaretto Chicken	20

	Chicken Thighs	21
	Shredded Barbecue Chicken	22
	Chicken Stew	23
	Lemon Pepper Chicken	24
	Italian Ranch Chicken	25
	Chicken with Wild Rice	26
	Fast Chicken Dinner	27
	Chicken with Pineapple	28
	Garlic Chicken	29
	Soy Honey Chicken	30
	Ritz Chicken Casserole	31
	Chicken Noodle Soup	32
	Crock-Pot Chicken Rice Soup	33
Chapter 3	Beef Dinners	35
	Ground Beef Cabbage Stew	35
	Beef Stew with Vegetables	37
	Easy Chili	38
	Beef Stroganoff	39
	Chinese Beef and Broccoli	40
	Goulash	41

Chili Pie	42
Spicy Beef	43
Beef Fajitas	44
Fast Lasagna	45
Beef and Corn Soup	46
Meatballs	47
Beef Tips	48
Easy Meatloaf	49
Creamy Beef Bake	50
Cheese and Beef Ravioli	51
Mongolian Beef	52
Calico Beans	53
Pepperoncini Pot Roast	54
Beefy Macaroni and Cheese	55
Cowboy Casserole	56
Sloppy Joes	57
Cheeseburger Soup	58
Taco Soup	59
Three-Ingredient Pot Roast	60
Stuffed Pepper Skillet	61

	Chili Mac	62
Chapter 4	Seafood Dinners	63
	Potato and Shrimp Chowder	63
	Beans with Tuna	65
	Tuna Noodle Casserole	66
	Shrimp Casserole	67
	Veggie and Shrimp Ramen Noodles	68
	Clam Chowder	69
	Tilapia with Spinach	70
	Garlic Shrimp Casserole	71
	One-Pan Baked Salmon	72
	One-Dish Italian Halibut	73
Chapter 5	Pork and Turkey Dinners	75
	Hungarian Pea Stew	75
	Sweet Pork Medallions	77
	Barbecued Pork Strips	78
	Baked Beans with Salt Pork	79
	Chunky Turkey Chili	80
	Turkey Breast	81
	Apple Cider Pork	82

	Spicy Pork Chops	83
	Pork Chops with Rice	84
	Ranch Pork Chops	85
	Sweet Pork Chops	86
	Cheesy Pork Chops	87
	Creamy Pork Chops	88
	Tuscan Pork Chops	89
	Bleu Cheese Chops	90
	Turkey Casserole	91
	Turkey and Broccoli Casserole	92
Chapter 6	Vegetarian Dinners and Sides	93
	Crock-Pot Eggplant	93
	Brown Potato Soup	95
	Mexican Dip	96
	Barbecue Bean Soup	97
	Baked Pineapple Stuffing	98
	Cheesy Hash Browns	99
	Ginger Potato Casserole	100
	Mushroom Macaroni	101
	Tofu Fajitas	102

	Red Beans and Rice	103
	Spinach Ravioli Bake	104
	Garlic and Cheese Potatoes	105
	Coconut Rice	106
	Cheesy Bread Rolls	107
	Lemon and Herb Orzo	108
	Lentil Soup	109
	Cheese Pizza	110
	Cheese Tortellini	111
	Veggie Casserole	112
Chapter 7	Bonus Desserts	113
	Chocolate Pudding Cake	113
	Apple Dump Cake	115
	Cherry Dump Cake	116
	Banana Split Dump Cake	117
	Pumpkin Dump Cake	118
A Little Food For Thought...		119

Introduction

Have you ever wondered what your life would be like if you could eat healthy home-cooked meals without slaving in the kitchen every night?

How would you like to spend more time with your family than your oven?

Or have you ever thought about all the money you could save if you stopped reaching for the take-out menu after a long day at the office?

If you want to be able to make a delicious homemade meal for your family every night without spending your entire evening in the kitchen, then this book can help show you how this is not just possible, but easy.

Dump Dinners: 101 Easy, Delicious, and Healthy Meals Put Together in 30 Minutes or Less! reveals 101 simple yet delicious meals that can be thrown together in the blink of an eye, leaving you with more money in your pocket and more memories with your family.

The best part is that you don't need to be a great cook to make these meals. With easy-to-get ingredients and simple instructions, you'll be in charge of your kitchen in no time.

One great advantage to this cooking technique is that once you get a few recipes under your belt, it will become easier to look into your refrigerator and pantry and see how a dump dinner can come together. You will know what to shop for and how to organize your kitchen so that dinner comes together even faster than you ever imagined.

In **Dump Dinners: 101 Easy, Delicious, and Healthy Meals Put Together in 30 Minutes or Less!** you will learn some of the best recipes out there that have been put together by people just like you. They have busy schedules but still want to provide their families with a balanced diet. You will be left wondering why you haven't been cooking this way forever.

So let's head to the kitchen but there's no need to put on an apron. You won't be in there very long!

Chapter 1
What's For Dinner?

It's no secret that we are all busy people these days. Between work, school, the kids' sports, taking the dog for a walk, folding the laundry and keeping the house from looking like a science experiment, how in the world are you supposed to make a healthy and delicious meal?

It seems like there are two options. Either spend your evening in the kitchen prepping, chopping, grilling, baking, and cleaning, or reach for the phone and the take-out menu. But here's where we are wrong. There's a third option that is easy and affordable. Try a dump dinner!

What? Never heard of it? Despite the name, a dump dinner is a delicious and quick method of cooking that leaves you with more time in the evening to relax and spend time with your family. The concept is simple. You gather all of your ingredients and simply dump them into a casserole dish, a crock-pot or a large pot on the stove. Before you know it, dinner is served!

Here's a few tips and tricks to keep your dump dinner experience running smoothly.

Make a List

If you really want to embrace the dump dinner way of cooking, staying organized and prepared is crucial. There's nothing worse than having to make a trip to the store for one ingredient that you forgot. Try to get in the habit of planning your weekly dump dinners and making a list of ingredients. Ideally, you will eventually learn the best ingredients to keep on hand and have many of these items stocked up. Cross off any ingredients that you already have and you are left with your grocery list. One trip will get you everything that you need for a week (or more, depending on your planning) of homemade quick dinners.

Chop Veggies Right Away

If you buy your vegetables fresh, spend some time when you get home chopping them all. You can do it by hand of course but if you really want to speed things up, invest in a chopper. Separate the vegetables into either half cup or full cup servings and place them in a bag to be frozen. Some vegetables freeze better than others. Chances are, if you can buy them frozen you can freeze them yourself. That leads to the next part of this tip: if you don't want to chop your vegetables, simply buy them frozen.

Stock Up

Sometimes you find yourself with everything to make a dump dinner except for one ingredient. This will get easier as you go but you will find that there are some ingredients that you go through faster than others. Make a note of this and keep extra of this ingredient on hand.

Precook Meat

In most cases, buying in bulk can help save you money. If

you practice this money saving technique, try cooking all of your meat for the week when you get home. Brown all of your ground beef and drain it. Cook all of your chicken and cube or shred it. Make meatballs or cook Italian sausage for a lasagna. Depending on when you are going to use the meat in a dump dinner, keep it in the refrigerator or freeze it. By doing all of your cooking at once, putting together dump dinners will be even quicker when all you have to do is reach for a bag of chicken or precooked meatballs.

Frozen Dinners

If you are making one dump dinner, spend a little extra time making two and freeze the second one. This works really well for most casseroles and crock-pot meals. Remember that certain dairy products don't freeze well, such as sour cream. Adjust recipes accordingly if you plan on freezing them. Crock-pot meals can be placed in a large freezer bag. Save room by freezing them flat. Make sure to label and date everything. Soups, stews and chili freeze well, too. Make a double batch, freeze half and you have a quick dinner for the future.

If you're ready, let's dive into the world of dump dinners. It won't take long to get the hang of it and you will be left with only one question; who decided that making dinner required so much work for so long?

Chapter 2
Chicken Dinners

Chicken is always a great 'go-to' meat for dinner. It's healthy, affordable, and offers so many different combinations that are sure to satisfy any taste palate. Most chicken recipes are great reheated so don't be afraid to make extra for leftovers the next day.

Creamy Chicken Casserole

Quick and easy, this casserole is hearty and great for a cold day. Canned chicken can be used or leftover shredded chicken is a great money saving option.

Ingredients:

2 cans cream of chicken soup
8 ounces sour cream
1 ¾ cups milk, divided
6-8 cups diced chicken, cooked
1 teaspoon salt
½ teaspoon pepper
¾ cup Bisquick

¼ cup cornmeal
1 egg
8 ounces shredded Cheddar cheese

Directions:

Preheat oven to 375 degrees Fahrenheit. Combine the soup, sour cream, and 1 cup of milk together in a large bowl, mixing well. Stir in the chicken, salt, and pepper. Pour the mixture into a 9 x 13 baking dish. In a separate bowl, whisk the baking mix, cornmeal, egg, and remaining milk together. Place on top of chicken mixture using a spoon. Sprinkle the casserole with cheese. Bake for 30-35 minutes or until edges are golden brown and the entire casserole is hot.

Italian Chicken and Rice

Italian dishes are a favorite of many, including kids. This dish can be easily prepared during the day and ready to go in the oven when it's dinner time.

Ingredients:

2 cups marinara sauce
1 can (15 ounces) Italian-seasoned diced tomatoes (undrained)
1 cup uncooked long grain white rice
1 ½ pounds skinless, boneless chicken breast (uncooked)
1 teaspoon Italian seasoning
½ cup shredded mozzarella cheese
¼ cup grated Parmesan cheese
2 tablespoons chopped fresh parsley (optional)

Directions:

Preheat oven to 375 degrees Fahrenheit. Stir the marinara sauce, tomatoes, and rice together in a 9 x 13 baking dish. Place the chicken breasts on top. Sprinkle the chicken with Italian seasoning and cover the dish tightly with aluminum foil. Make sure that it is tight so that steam cannot escape, otherwise the rice won't cook. Bake for 45 minutes or until the chicken is cooked all the way and the rice is soft. Remove the foil and sprinkle with the cheeses. Continue baking for 5 more minutes or until the cheese is melted. If desired, garnish with parsley before serving.

Mexican Chicken Lasagna

This casserole comes together quickly and is sure to please a crowd. Feel free to get creative with toppings, like sour cream, chopped tomatoes or pickled jalapeno slices.

Ingredients:

1 can cream of mushroom soup
1 can cream of chicken soup
3 cups chicken, chopped and cooked
1 can mild Ro-Tel
1 cup frozen corn
1 can nacho cheese
4 large, burrito-style flour tortillas
2 cups Mexican shredded cheese blend
1 can black beans, rinsed
¼ cup fresh cilantro, chopped

Directions:

Preheat oven to 175 degrees Fahrenheit. Mix together cooked chicken, both cream soups, nacho cheese, Ro-Tel, and cilantro in a large bowl. Place 1 cup of the mixture into a greased casserole dish. Alternate layers of tortillas, cheese, beans, and the mixture until all ingredients have been used. Cover the dish with aluminum foil and bake for 20 minutes. Uncover and continue baking until fully heated, about 10 more minutes. Add desired garnishes and serve.

Creamy Peanut Chicken

This Asian-inspired dish pairs great with simple instant white rice. For an added kick, try adding some crushed red pepper to the sauce.

Ingredients:

2 tablespoons oil
1 tablespoon soy sauce
3 tablespoons creamy peanut butter
3 tablespoons ketchup
4 chicken breasts

Directions:

Place the chicken in the bottom of a crock-pot. Mix all ingredients together in a bowl and pour over the chicken. Cook for 8 to 10 hours on low.

Chicken Mushroom Casserole

Chicken and mushrooms are a classic pair. While canned mushrooms will work just fine, try different kinds of fresh mushrooms to mix it up.

Ingredients:

1 onion, chopped
3 cups sliced mushrooms
2 tablespoons coconut oil
½ teaspoon salt
¼ teaspoon ground black pepper
½ teaspoon minced garlic
2 large chicken breasts with skin on

Directions:

Oil a casserole dish with the coconut oil. Place the chicken breasts in. Mix all other ingredients together and pour over the chicken. Cover and bake for 1 ½ hours at 400 degrees Fahrenheit.

Spicy Lime Chicken

Change the amount of spices depending on your desired level of heat. This is a great recipe to double and freeze if you have the time.

Ingredients:

4-6 boneless, skinless chicken breasts
1 tablespoon olive oil
1 tablespoon lime juice
2 tablespoons chili powder
1 teaspoon cayenne
salt and pepper to taste

Directions:

Preheat the oven to 350 degrees Fahrenheit. Mix all of the ingredients in a large baking dish. Make sure that all sides of the chicken are covered in the mixture. Bake for 30-60 minutes or until the chicken is done and juices run clear.

Easiest Chicken Casserole

From cabinet to table in under half an hour, this casserole is about as easy as they come. Leftover chicken can be substituted.

Ingredients:

1 (5 ounce) can chunk chicken, drained
1 can cream of chicken soup
1 can chicken noodle soup
1 can chow mein noodles

Directions:

Preheat oven to 350 degrees Fahrenheit. Mix all of the ingredients together in a casserole dish. Bake for 20 minutes.

Chicken, Tomato, and Rice Casserole

This simple dish is incredibly economical and yet tasty. Most of the time is spent simmering the dish, leaving you free to catch up on kitchen chores while it cooks.

Ingredients:

4 boneless, skinless chicken breasts
3 cups water
3 cups chicken stock
2 (15 ounce) cans tomato sauce
1 large onion, chopped
2 cups long grain rice, rinsed
salt and pepper to taste

Directions:

Mix all ingredients except for the rice in a large pot. Bring to a boil over medium-high heat. Cover and cook for 30 minutes. Mix in the rice and continue cooking for another 20 minutes or until the rice has soaked in most of the liquid.

Honey Onion Ginger Chicken

There's nothing boring going on in this dinner. Picky eaters will unite around the dinner table with this great combination of flavors.

Ingredients:

1 ½ pounds chicken pieces
4 tablespoons chopped onion
1 ½ tablespoons honey
1 tablespoon soy sauce
1 tablespoon minced ginger
2 tablespoons sherry
¼ cup chives

Directions:

Preheat the oven to 350 degrees Fahrenheit. Mix all ingredients together in a bowl, making sure that chicken is coated. Pour into a 9 x 13 baking dish and cook until the chicken is no longer pink and juices run clear, anywhere from 30-60 minutes depending on the size of the chicken.

Monterey Jack Chicken and Rice Casserole

Cheese, chicken, and rice are casserole staples. Enjoy this quick dish on a relaxing evening in.

Ingredients:

2 cups cooked rice
2 cups shredded Monterey Jack cheese
2 cups cooked, shredded chicken breast
1 cup chicken broth
12 ounces evaporated milk
2 large eggs, slightly beaten
1 tablespoon onion powder
2 tablespoons dried basil
½ teaspoon salt
2 tablespoons melted butter
1 tablespoon finely diced jalapenos

Directions:

Preheat oven to 375 degrees Fahrenheit. Lightly grease a 2 quart-casserole dish. Combine the rice, cheese, chicken, chicken broth, evaporated milk, onion powder, eggs, basil, butter, and jalapenos in prepared casserole dish. Stir well. Bake, uncovered, for 30 minutes.

All-in-One Chicken Dinner

This meal makes you individual portions of chicken and veggies. Perfect for nights when everyone has to eat at different times due to schedule conflicts.

Ingredients:

8 boneless, skinless chicken breasts
½ teaspoon salt
1 teaspoon Italian seasoning
½ teaspoon tarragon
6 potatoes, sliced
2 cups sliced carrots

Directions:

Preheat oven to 400 degrees Fahrenheit. Spray 8 large pieces of foil with cooking spray. In each piece of foil, place 1 piece of chicken and even portions of carrots and potatoes. Season each piece of chicken. Wrap tightly in the foil and bake for 30-35 minutes.

General Tsao's Chicken

No need to ever order take-out again with this dish. Add more red pepper if you want a little more heat.

Ingredients:

4 boneless skinless chicken breasts
½ cup water
3 tablespoons hoisen sauce
2 tablespoons soy sauce
½ cup brown sugar
3 tablespoons ketchup
¼ teaspoon dry ginger
½ teaspoon crushed red pepper
1 tablespoon cornstarch

Directions:

Mix the sugar, sauces, ketchup, ginger, and red pepper in a bowl. Place the chicken in a crock-pot. Pour the mixture over the chicken and cook on low for 6 hours. Remove the chicken and cut into bite-sized pieces. Stir the cornstarch into the sauce. Replace the chicken and cook for 15 more minutes. Serve over rice if desired.

Chicken and Stuffing

Make this before leaving the house in the morning. When you come home, the house will smell like you've been slaving over the stove all day.

Ingredients:

4-6 boneless skinless chicken breasts
1 small box Stove Top Stuffing for chicken
1 (10 ounce) package frozen chopped broccoli, thawed
1 can broccoli with cheese soup
½ cup chicken broth

Directions:

Place the chicken in the bottom of a crock-pot. Mix all other ingredients together in a bowl and pour over the chicken. Cook on low for 6 to 7 hours.

Apricot Chicken

Perfect for a summer night, this dish is unbelievably fast to put together. Enjoy with fresh veggies or salad.

Ingredients:

1/3 cup apricot preserves
1/3 cup Russian dressing
½ envelope onion soup mix
6 frozen chicken breasts

Directions:

Place the chicken in the bottom of a crock-pot. Mix all other ingredients together and pour over the chicken Cook on low 5 to 6 hours.

Amaretto Chicken

Don't let the name fool you. Even kids can enjoy this tasty chicken meal that comes together in minutes.

Ingredients:

4 to 6 boneless skinless chicken breasts
½ cup flour
1 teaspoon curry powder
1 teaspoon garlic powder
¼ teaspoon salt
¼ teaspoon pepper
1 tablespoon vegetable oil
1 can cream of mushroom soup
1 (4 ounce or more) can mushrooms
¼ cup amaretto
1 teaspoon Kitchen Bouquet
2 tablespoons lemon juice

Directions:

Mix flour, curry powder, garlic powder, salt, and pepper in a bag. Rinse chicken and add to bag. Shake to coat. Place the coated chicken into a crock-pot. Mix remaining ingredients together and pour over chicken. Cover and cook on low for 6 to 8 hours. Serve over rice if desired.

Chicken Thighs

Chicken thighs are often the most affordable part of a chicken but sometimes it's hard to come up with new ways to flavor them. Look no more.

Ingredients:

8 chicken thighs
salt and pepper to taste
12 ounces apricot jam
2 tablespoons honey
2 tablespoons Dijon mustard

Directions:

Place all ingredients in a crock-pot and toss well to coat. Cook on low for 5 to 6 hours.

Shredded Barbecue Chicken

This recipe is great for leftover chicken. Double or triple the recipe for parties or when you have to feed a crowd.

Ingredients:

2 pounds shredded chicken
1 jar barbecue sauce

Directions:

Place ingredients in a crock-pot. Cover and cook on low for 6 to 8 hours. Serve over rice or on hamburger buns.

Chicken Stew

This stew will warm you up from the inside out. It's hearty and flavorful and comes together in a flash.

Ingredients:

1 tablespoon olive oil
6 slices bacon, diced
8 ounces mushrooms, sliced
1 red bell pepper, chopped
1 green bell pepper, chopped
6 bunch green onions, sliced
4 chicken breast halves, boneless, cut into 1 inch chunks
4 ounces sliced ripe olives
2 tablespoon balsamic vinegar
1 small can tomato paste
1 (14.5 ounce) can tomatoes
¼ cup chicken broth
½ teaspoon dried ground marjoram
½ teaspoon salt
¼ teaspoon pepper

Directions:

Add olive oil to crock-pot. Spread bacon over the bottom. Add the mushrooms, bell peppers and green onions. Add chicken on top. Add the remaining ingredients. Cover and cook for 8 to 10 hours on low. Stir occasionally.

Lemon Pepper Chicken

Lemon and pepper are a simple concept that is taken to a new level in this recipe. Enjoy over rice or with sautéed vegetables.

Ingredients:

½ teaspoon grated lemon peel
2 cloves garlic, minced
¼ cup lemon juice
1 teaspoon pepper
1 tablespoon vegetable oil
¼ teaspoon salt
1 ½ pounds chicken pieces

Directions:

Preheat oven to 350 degrees Fahrenheit. Stir all ingredients together, making sure to coat the chicken. Bake for 30 minutes or until chicken is no longer pink and juices run clear.

Italian Ranch Chicken

Everyone loves Ranch and this dish has just enough of the flavor to keep people asking for seconds. If you don't have a packet of seasoning, it's easy to make your own version.

Ingredients:

4-6 chicken breasts
½ a small bottle of Italian dressing
1 packet of dry Ranch seasoning
½ cup water
½ tablespoon minced garlic
½ tablespoon chili powder
½ tablespoon ground cumin

Directions:

Mix all ingredients together in a crock-pot, stirring well. Cook on low for 4 to 6 hours.

Chicken with Wild Rice

A perfect Sunday night meal, this dinner is a keeper. Impress family or guests with this sophisticated skillet to casserole meal.

Ingredients:

2 (6 ounce) packages long grain and wild rice mix
8 chicken breast halves
5 tablespoons butter, divided
1 sweet red pepper, chopped
2 (4 ½ ounce) jars sliced mushrooms, drained

Directions:

Preheat oven to 350 degrees Fahrenheit. Cook the rice according to package directions. Melt 3 tablespoons of butter and sauté the chicken for 7 minutes on each side. Transfer to a platter to keep warm. Melt the rest of the butter in the skillet and sauté the red pepper. Add the mushrooms and heat thoroughly. Combine with the rice. Pour the mixture in the bottom of a casserole dish and place chicken on top. Bake for 30 minutes or until chicken is finished cooking.

Fast Chicken Dinner

Do you only have four minutes to make dinner? Then this is the recipe for you. Make before running errands or picking up the kids from school and dinner will be ready when you are.

Ingredients:

4 chicken breasts
½ cup ketchup
¼ cup water
¼ cup packed brown sugar
3 tablespoons dry onion soup mix

Directions:

Place the chicken in the bottom of a crock-pot. Mix other ingredients together and pour over chicken. Cover and cook on low for 4 to 6 hours.

Chicken with Pineapple

Orange juice and pineapple give this chicken dish a light and tropical flavor. Make a second batch and freeze in a sealable bag for an even easier second dinner.

Ingredients:

4 chicken breasts
1 (8 ounce) can pineapple chunks, undrained
¼ cup packed brown sugar
½ teaspoon nutmeg
1/3 cup orange juice
½ cup raisins

Directions:

Place the chicken in the bottom of a crock-pot. Mix other ingredients together and pour over chicken. Cover and cook for 4 to 6 hours.

Garlic Chicken

A little garlic never hurt anyone. Get your garlic fix with this quick crock-pot meal.

Ingredients:

4 chicken breasts
2-3 cloves garlic, minced
4 tablespoons olive oil
2 tablespoons fresh chopped parsley
3 tablespoons lemon juice
¼ teaspoon pepper

Directions:

Place the chicken in the bottom of a crock-pot. Mix all ingredients together in a bowl and pour over the chicken. Cook for 4 to 6 hours on low.

Soy Honey Chicken

Try something new tonight! This sweet chicken dish will disappear before your eyes once it hits the table.

Ingredients:

½ cup ketchup
¼ cup melted honey
¼ cup soy sauce
2 tablespoons lemon juice
4 chicken breasts

Directions:

Place the chicken in the bottom of a crock-pot. Mix all ingredients together in a bowl and pour over the chicken. Cook for 4 to 6 hours on low.

Ritz Chicken Casserole

The classic cracker adds a fun crunch to this casserole. Try different flavored crackers for a twist.

Ingredients:

3 chicken breasts, cooked and diced
16 ounce egg noodles, cooked
24 ounces sour cream
2 cans cream of chicken soup
8 ounces shredded Cheddar cheese
8 ounces shredded mozzarella cheese
1 sleeve Ritz crackers, crushed
¼ cup margarine, melted

Directions:

Preheat oven to 350 degrees Fahrenheit. Mix the chicken, sour cream, soup, and cheese in a bowl. Toss in the noodles and stir gently to coat. Pour into a baking dish. Sprinkle with crackers and drizzle with margarine. Bake for 30 minutes.

Chicken Noodle Soup

It's classic but it's delicious. Freeze extras for when you need a little pick me up.

Ingredients:

2 (32 ounce) cartons chicken stock
½ teaspoon poultry seasoning
½ teaspoon garlic powder
½ teaspoon onion powder
1 pound boneless chicken
1 cup diced carrots
½ cup diced celery
1 can cream of chicken soup
3 cups water
3 cups egg noodles, uncooked
salt and pepper to taste

Directions:

Pour the chicken stock into a large pot. Add the chicken, followed by the seasonings. Stir well. Cover and cook on high for 25 minutes or until chicken is cooked. Remove chicken and shred. Place back in pot and add veggies. Stir in cream of chicken soup and add the water. Add noodles and stir. Cover and cook on medium for about 20 minutes or until vegetables are tender. Add salt and pepper to taste.

Crock-Pot Chicken Rice Soup

Perfect for a cold winter day, this soup cooks while you're out playing. Serve with toasted bread for a filling meal.

Ingredients:

3 (14 ½ ounce) cans chicken broth
2 pounds boneless, skinless chicken breasts, cut into bite-sized pieces
2 cups water
1 cup sliced celery
1 cup diced carrot
1 (6 ounce) package long grain and wild rice blend
½ cup chopped onion
½ teaspoon ground black pepper
1 teaspoon dried parsley flakes

Directions:

Mix all ingredients in a crock-pot. Stir well. Cover and cook on low for 6 to 7 hours or on high for 4 to 5 hours.

Chapter 3: Beef Dinners

Beef is a staple in most dinners. This chapter has a wide variety of different types of beef to incorporate into your meals.

Ground Beef Cabbage Stew

This stew can be made quickly and it serves plenty. It's great for last-minute company.

Ingredients:

1 ½ pounds ground beef
1 cup beef stock
1 onion, chopped
1 bay leaf
¼ teaspoon pepper
2 celery ribs, sliced
4 cups cabbage, shredded
1 carrot, sliced
1 cup tomato paste
¼ teaspoon salt

Directions:

Brown ground meat in a large pot. Add the beef stock, onion, pepper, bay leaf, celery, cabbage and carrot. Cover and simmer until vegetables are tender. Mix in tomato paste and salt and continue to simmer uncovered for 20 minutes.

Beef Stew with Vegetables

This is about as traditional as it gets. Easy to make and it tastes just like Grandma's version.

Ingredients:

1 ½ cups chopped carrots
1 cup chopped onion
2 tablespoons coconut oil
1 ½ cups green peas
4 cups beef stock
½ teaspoon salt
¼ teaspoon ground black pepper
½ teaspoon minced garlic
4 pounds boneless chuck roast

Directions:

Melt the coconut oil in a large pot and add the onions. Cook until tender and then add all other ingredients. Stir well. Cover and cook on low heat for 2 hours. Add cornstarch mixed with water if needed to thicken to desired consistency.

Easy Chili

Every cook needs a quick chili recipe and this is it. It's perfect for football season or any fall day. Serve with sour cream, cheese or jalapenos as garnish.

Ingredients:

1 pound ground beef
1 (14.5) can diced tomatoes and green chilies, undrained
2 (15 ounce) cans chili beans
1 (11.5) can spicy vegetable juice
1 onion, chopped
1 teaspoon cumin
1 teaspoon garlic powder
salt and pepper to taste

Directions:

Brown the beef in a skillet. Once cooked, combine with all other ingredients in a slow cooker. Cover and cook on low for 4 to 6 hours.

Beef Stroganoff

A creamy and filling meal, this comes together fast and easy. Try over rice or toast for a change.

Ingredients:

2 pounds stew meat (cut into bite-size pieces)
1 can mushrooms
1 package onion soup mix
1 can cream of mushroom soup
1 can ginger ale
2 tablespoons corn starch
8 ounces sour cream at room temperature
1 package egg noodles

Directions:

Place frozen stew meat in a crock-pot. Add mushrooms, onion soup mix, cream of mushroom soup, and ginger ale. Cook on high for 4 to 5 hours or on low for 6 to 7 hours, stirring occasionally. During the last hour, mix corn starch with a small amount of water and add it to the crock-pot to thicken the mixture. Add sour cream to taste. When ready to serve, cook egg noodles according to package directions and spoon beef mixture over the noodles.

Chinese Beef and Broccoli

This tastes just like the restaurant version but without the bill. Add other vegetables as desired.

Ingredients:

1 pound beef chuck roast, cut into thin strips
1 cup beef broth
½ cup soy sauce
1/3 cup brown sugar
1 tablespoon sesame oil
3 garlic cloves, minced
2 tablespoons cornstarch
2 tablespoons water
2 cups frozen broccoli
rice, for serving

Directions:

In a crock-pot, whisk together the beef broth, soy sauce, brown sugar, sesame oil, and garlic. Add the beef and stir to coat. Cook on low for 6 hours. Whisk together the cornstarch and water in a small bowl and add to the crock-pot. Stir well and continue cooking for 30 minutes. Add broccoli and stir. Meal is ready once the broccoli is cooked, only a few minutes. Serve over prepared rice, if desired.

Goulash

Try this version of a Hungarian classic. It's an easy one-pot meal that the whole family will enjoy.

Ingredients:

1 ½ pounds beef round steak, cut into chunks
2 potatoes, peeled and quartered
2 onions, chopped
4 carrots, chopped
2 tomatoes, chopped
2 cups beef broth
1 ½ cups water
¼ cup butter
1 teaspoon paprika
½ teaspoon black pepper

Directions:

Melt the butter in a large pot over high heat. Add the steak and onions. Cook for a few minutes, until the meat is browned. Add the rest of the ingredients, minus the tomatoes, cover and reduce heat to low. Simmer for 45 minutes. Add the tomatoes and continue to simmer, uncovered, for 25 to 30 minutes or until the beef is tender and the sauce has thickened.

Chili Pie

Feel free to save some time by using leftover chili in this recipe. Adjust spices to taste.

Ingredients:

1 pound lean ground beef
1 can diced tomatoes, drained
1 onion, chopped
1 package chili seasoning mix
1 can sliced ripe olives, drained
1 cup shredded Cheddar cheese, divided
½ cup original Bisquick mix
1 cup milk
2 eggs
chopped tomato, red onion, jalapeno, and sour cream for garnish, if desired

Directions:

Preheat oven to 400 degrees Fahrenheit. Spray the bottom of a 9" glass pie pan and set aside. Cook the ground beef in a skillet over medium heat. Drain and then stir in the tomatoes, onion, and chili seasoning mix. Spread in the pie pan. Sprinkle with a layer of olives and a ½ cup of cheese. In a medium bowl, stir the Bisquick, milk, and eggs with a whisk until blended. Pour into the pie pan. Bake for 30 minutes. Top with remaining cheese and bake for another couple of minutes until melted. Serve with desired toppings.

Spicy Beef

If you're looking for something spicy, this is it. Add more hot sauce if you want but proceed with caution.

Ingredients:

4 pound pot roast, boneless and trimmed
1 onion, sliced
3 potatoes, peeled and sliced
1 tablespoon mustard
1 tablespoon hot sauce
1 tablespoon Worcestershire sauce
2 tablespoons flour
1 teaspoon vinegar
1 teaspoon sugar

Directions:

Mix the flour, mustard, chili sauce, Worcestershire sauce, vinegar, and sugar. Spread the mixture on top of the roast. Place the potatoes and onions on the bottom of a crock-pot and then place the roast on top. Cover and cook on high for 5 to 6 hours or on low for 10 to 12 hours.

Beef Fajitas

Everyone loves fajitas and with this recipe you can have them whenever you want. To save more time, buy a fajita kit with the beef and vegetables ready to go.

Ingredients:

1 ½ pound flank steak, trimmed and cut into 5 to 7 pieces
1 bell pepper, chopped
1 red onion, chopped
2 jalapeno peppers, chopped
½ tablespoon parsley
1 teaspoon cumin
1 teaspoon garlic powder
1 teaspoon chili powder
1 teaspoon coriander
¼ teaspoon salt
1 (8 ounce) can stewed tomatoes
12 7-inch tortillas

Directions:

Combine all of the ingredients, minus the tortillas, in a crock-pot. Cover and cook on low for 8 to 10 hours or on high for 4 to 5 hours. Shred the beef and stir back in the crock-pot.

Fast Lasagna

If you knew lasagna could be this easy you wouldn't have avoided it so much. Substitute the cottage cheese for Ricotta if desired.

Ingredients:

1 pound ground beef
1 (48 ounce) jar pasta sauce
1 (16 ounce) package lasagna noodles
2 eggs, beaten
1 (24 ounce) carton small curd cottage cheese
4 cups shredded mozzarella cheese

Directions:

Preheat the oven to 350 degrees Fahrenheit. Brown the beef and drain. Stir in the pasta sauce and stir to coat. In a separate bowl, combine the egg and cottage cheese. Place 1/3 of the meat mixture on the bottom of a 9 x 13 inch baking dish. Cover with a double layer of uncooked lasagna noodles. Follow with ½ of the cottage cheese mixture. Repeat this process twice. Top with the mozzarella cheese. Bake for 1 hour and 15 minutes or until the noodles are tender.

Beef and Corn Soup

This soup is easy to make but tastes like it isn't. Mix and match vegetables if you don't have everything.

Ingredients:

1 pound ground beef
1 (14 ½ ounce) can corn
1 (14 ½ ounce) can green beans
1 (14 ½ ounce) can carrots
1 (14 ½ ounce) can green peas
1 (15 ounce) can stewed tomatoes
4 beef bouillon cubes
4 potatoes, peeled and chopped
3 garlic cloves, diced
water

Directions:

In a pot, brown the beef and garlic together. Start adding all of the vegetables, including the liquid. Add the potatoes and bouillon cubes. Add water as needed. Simmer for about 4 hours.

Meatballs

Make these meatballs as a meal by themselves or to add to other meals. They freeze easily.

Ingredients:

1 ½ pounds extra lean ground beef
1 cup dry breadcrumbs
½ cup egg substitute
1/3 cup chopped fresh parsley
2 tablespoons minced fresh onion
1/3 cup ketchup
2 tablespoons brown sugar
1 tablespoon lemon juice
16 ounces cranberry sauce
12 ounces chili sauce

Directions:

In a large bowl, mix together the ground beef, parsley, breadcrumbs, onion, and egg substitute. Form about 30 meatballs. In a crock-pot, mix together the ketchup, juice, sugar, and sauces. Stir very well. Gently place the meatballs in and cover. Cook for 8 to 10 hours on low.

Beef Tips

The beef in this recipe will melt in your mouth after cooking all day. Serve over mashed potatoes or rice.

Ingredients:

2 pounds beef, cubed
1 can cream of chicken soup
1 can cream of celery soup
3 tablespoons onion soup mix
½ soup can of water

Directions:

Spray the inside of a crock-pot with cooking spray. Mix all ingredients together and pour into the crock-pot. Cook on low for 6 to 8 hours or until the meat is tender.

Easy Meatloaf

Meatloaf doesn't have to be an all-day process. Make this the night before and start the crock-pot in the morning.

Ingredients:

1 ½ pounds ground chuck
1 egg, beaten
¼ cup milk
1 ½ teaspoon salt
2 slices bread, crumbed
½ onion, chopped
2 tablespoons chopped green pepper
2 tablespoons chopped celery
6 potatoes, cut up
ketchup to taste

Directions:

Mix egg, milk, salt, and breadcrumbs together. Allow to stand to soften. Mix the egg mixture with the ground chuck and chopped vegetables. Shape into a loaf and place in a crock-pot. Top with ketchup. Place the cut up potatoes around the sides of the loaf. Cover and cook on high for 1 hour and reduce heat to low. Continue cooking for 8-9 more hours.

Creamy Beef Bake

Noodles, beef, and creamy sauce come together perfectly in this dish. Serve with steamed vegetables for a full meal.

Ingredients:

8 ounce penne noodles, cooked
½ pound ground beef
½ onion, chopped
1 can fire roasted diced tomatoes
1 teaspoon dried oregano
1 tablespoon butter
2 garlic cloves, chopped
1 tablespoon flour
1 (12 ounce) can evaporated milk
8 ounces cream cheese, cut into chunks
1 teaspoon salt, divided
1 ½ cups shredded mozzarella cheese

Directions:

Preheat oven to 375 degrees Fahrenheit. In a saucepan, mix the tomatoes, beef, onion, oregano, and ½ teaspoon of salt and cook well. Heat butter in a separate skillet and cook the garlic. Lower the heat and stir in the flour. Mix in the milk, cream cheese, and the rest of the salt. Allow the mixture to thicken. Combine the meat, sauce, and noodles in a baking dish. Sprinkle with the cheese. Bake for 25 minutes or until bubbly.

Cheese and Beef Ravioli

It doesn't get much easier than this. Serve with garlic bread and salad and dinner is done.

Ingredients:

1 pound ground beef, cooked
25 ounces frozen ravioli
1 jar spaghetti sauce
1 cup shredded mozzarella cheese

Directions:

Dump the beef, ravioli and spaghetti in a crock-pot. Mix well. Cover and cook for 2-3 hours on high. Top with the mozzarella cheese, let melt and serve.

Mongolian Beef

This dish is great over rice or by itself. The meat is perfectly tender and the sauce has the perfect balance of taste.

Ingredients:

1 ½ pounds flank steak
¼ cup corn starch
2 tablespoons olive oil
½ teaspoon minced garlic
¾ cup soy sauce
¾ cup water
¾ cup brown sugar
½ cup shredded carrots
3 green onions, chopped

Directions:

Slice the steak into strips. Cover each piece in cornstarch. Mix the rest of the ingredients in a crock-pot and add the steak. Cook on high for 2 to 3 hours or on low for 4 to 5 hours. Serve over rice or noodles if desired.

Calico Beans

This dish gets its name from the different colored beans. Kids will love it and it tastes great as leftovers too.

Ingredients:

1 large can baked bean
1 regular can kidney beans
1 regular can butter beans
1 pound ground beef, browned
1 pound bacon, cooked and chopped
1 onion, chopped
½ cup dark brown sugar
¼ cup ketchup
¼ cup barbecue sauce

Directions:

Mix all ingredients together in a crock-pot. Cook on low for 2 to 4 hours.

Pepperoncini Pot Roast

Try this unique pot roast for something different. Serve over mashed potatoes or make sandwiches from the roast.

Ingredients:

2 to 3 pound lean pot roast
32 ounce jar pepperoncini
3 to 4 garlic cloves, chopped

Directions:

Place the roast into a crock-pot. Dump entire jar of peppers and liquid over the roast. Add garlic. Cover and cook on low for 8 to 10 hours.

Beefy Macaroni and Cheese

This recipe has a few extra steps but it is still quick and easy to make. Kids love the macaroni and cheese combination in this dish.

Ingredients:

1 ½ pounds lean ground beef
1 onion, chopped
1 envelope cheese sauce mix
¼ cup water
1 can cream of mushroom soup
1 (15 ounce) can stewed tomatoes
2 tablespoons tomato paste
1 cup shredded cheddar cheese
8 ounces macaroni, cooked

Directions:

Brown ground beef and onion. Add all other ingredients, except shredded cheese and macaroni, in a crock-pot. Add beef and onions. Cover and cook on low for 6 hours. Add cheese and macaroni. Continue cooking for 30 more minutes or until cheese has melted.

Cowboy Casserole

After a day of hard outdoor work, this meal hits the spot. Try any type of potato desired.

Ingredients:

1 ½ pounds ground chuck, browned and drained
1 onion, chopped
6 medium potatoes, sliced
1 can red beans
1 (8 ounce) can tomatoes mixed with 2 tablespoons flour
salt, pepper and garlic to taste

Directions:

Place chopped onion in the bottom of a crock-pot. Layer with browned ground beef, sliced potatoes, and beans. Spread tomatoes over all. Sprinkle with seasonings as desired. Cover and cook on low for 7 to 9 hours.

Sloppy Joes

It's one of America's favorites. Try this quick version of the classic sandwich.

Ingredients:

1 pound ground beef, browned
8 ounces tomato sauce
¼ cup brown sugar
1 cup barbecue sauce
½ cup ketchup
½ cup water
2 tablespoons cider vinegar
2 tablespoons mustard

Directions:

Place all ingredients in a crock-pot. Cover and cook on low for 4 to 6 hours, stirring occasionally.

Cheeseburger Soup

Yes, cheeseburger soup. It does taste as good as it sounds.

Ingredients:

1 pound ground beef, browned
¾ cup chopped onion
¾ cup shredded carrots
¾ cup diced celery
1 teaspoon dried basil
1 teaspoon dried parsley flakes
4 tablespoons butter, divided
3 cups chicken broth
4 cups peeled and diced potatoes
¼ cup all-purpose flour
2 cups shredded Cheddar cheese
1 ½ cups milk
¾ teaspoon salt
½ teaspoon pepper
¼ cup sour cream

Directions:

In a saucepan, melt one tablespoon of butter and cook onion, shredded carrots, parsley flakes, basil, and celery. Add the broth, potatoes, and ground beef. Bring to a boil. Reduce heat and simmer 10 to 12 minutes. In a separate skillet, melt the remaining butter and add the flour. Cook for 3 to 5 minutes. Add to the soup and stir. Reduce heat to low and stir in the cheese, milk, salt, and pepper. Cook until cheese has melted. Remove from heat and stir in sour cream.

Taco Soup

The hardest part about this recipe is opening up all the cans. But once you crack open that last one, dinner's made.

Ingredients:

1 pound ground beef, browned
1 (15 ounce) can black beans, drained and rinsed
1 (15 ounce) can pinto beans, drained and rinsed
1 (14.5 ounce) can petite diced tomatoes, drained
1 (15.25 ounce) can sweet corn, drained
1 can cream of chicken soup
1 can green enchilada sauce
1 (14 ounce) can chicken broth
1 packet taco seasoning

Directions:

Mix all ingredients together in a large pot. Heat until warm, stirring occasionally.

Three-Ingredient Pot Roast

Any cola brand will do in this recipe. It keeps the roast unbelievably moist.

Ingredients:

3 pound roast
1 package pot roast seasoning
1 package Au Jus mix
1 can cola

Directions:

Place the roast in a crock-pot. Sprinkle with seasonings and pour on the cola. Cover and cook for 8 hours on low, adding water if needed.

Stuffed Pepper Skillet

Don't spend your night stuffing vegetables. Make this quick casserole version that tastes just as great.

Ingredients:

1 pound extra-lean ground beef
½ cup diced onion
3 cloves garlic, minced
2 cups diced bell pepper
½ teaspoon salt
¼ teaspoon pepper
1 (14.5 ounce) can diced tomatoes, undrained
2 cups beef broth
8 ounces tomato sauce
1 tablespoon soy sauce
1 teaspoon Italian seasonings
1 cup instant white rice, uncooked
1 ½ cups shredded Cheddar cheese

Directions:

Brown the ground beef, garlic, and onions in a pan. Add peppers, salt, and pepper. Cook for 5 minutes. Reduce heat and add tomatoes, broth, tomato sauce, soy sauce, and Italian seasoning. Stir well. Bring to a boil and then add rice. Reduce heat to low. Cover and simmer for 25 minutes. Remove from heat and sprinkle on cheese. Serve immediately.

Chili Mac

This classic dish will please everyone at the table. Adjust the spices if needed to keep kids happy.

Ingredients:

1 pound ground beef
1 onion, diced
2 tablespoons garlic paste
2 cans chicken broth
1 (14.5 ounce) can diced tomatoes
½ can white kidney beans, drained and rinsed
½ can kidney beans, drained and rinsed
2 teaspoons chili powder
1 ½ teaspoons cumin
½ teaspoon season salt
¼ teaspoon ground pepper
10 ounces uncooked macaroni
2 cups shredded Cheddar cheese

Directions:

In a large pot, cook ground beef and onion until ground beef is no longer pink. Add garlic and cook for 2 more minutes. Add chicken broth, tomatoes, white kidney beans, kidney beans, chili powder, cumin, salt, and pepper. Mix well and bring to a boil. Add pasta and cook for 1 to 15 minutes or until pasta is cooked through. Stir as needed. When most of the liquid has been absorbed, add cheese and mix well. Cook for 5 more minutes and serve.

Chapter 4: Seafood Dinners

Seafood doesn't have to be complicated. Here are some great quick and easy recipes for you to try.

Potato and Shrimp Chowder

This soup does have to simmer for a long time but it's worth it, promise! Feel free to use fresh shrimp, just cook them separately before adding them to the chowder.

Ingredients:

3 potatoes, peeled and diced
1 cup sliced celery with tops
1 onion, chopped
2 cups boiling water
¼ teaspoon pepper
1 can evaporated milk
8 ounces Cheddar cheese, shredded
4 ½ ounce can tiny shrimp, undrained
4 tablespoons dry sherry
salt to taste
parsley, if desired

Directions:

Place the potatoes, onion and celery in a crock-pot. Pour the boiling water in. Cover and cook for 12 hours on low, or until the potatoes are tender. Mix in the evaporated milk, cheese, shrimp, and pepper one hour before desired serving time. Just before serving, mix in sherry and salt. Serve with parsley, if desired.

Beans with Tuna

This recipe involves a little planning since you have to drain the beans overnight. But other than that, it comes together quickly.

Ingredients:

4 tablespoons olive oil
1 clove garlic, crushed
1 pound small white beans, soaked overnight and drained
2 cups chopped tomatoes
2 (6 ½ ounce) cans white tuna in water, drained and flaked
1 ½ teaspoons dried basil
salt and pepper to taste

Directions:

Sauté the garlic with the oil in pan. Remove garlic and discard. Combine the garlic flavored oil with the beans and water in a crock-pot. Cover and cook on high for 2 hours. Turn heat to low and cook for another 8 hours. Add remaining ingredients and cook on high for an additional 30 minutes.

Tuna Noodle Casserole

Every Mom's go-to casserole, this version is quick and painless. Substitute the tuna for chicken or turkey.

Ingredients:

4 ounces whole wheat noodles
3 tablespoons breadcrumbs
2 tablespoons butter
½ cup diced onion
1 ½ cups diced mushrooms
2 tablespoons four
1 teaspoon fresh thyme
½ teaspoon pepper
1 ½ cups milk
12 ounces canned tuna, drained
¼ cup shredded Swiss cheese
2 cups frozen peas and carrots

Directions:

Preheat oven to 350 degrees Fahrenheit. Grease an 8 x 10 baking dish. Cook the noodles according to package directions. Melt the butter in a saucepan. Once melted, cook the onions and mushrooms for a few minutes. Sprinkle the flour over the mixture and stir to combine. Cook for 1 minute. Add the thyme and pepper, then the milk. Stir until the mixture comes to a boil. Reduce heat and simmer for a few minutes more. Add the tuna, cheese, peas and carrots, and noodles. Stir well and transfer to baking dish. Top with breadcrumbs. Bake for 20 minutes or until bubbly.

Shrimp Casserole

Try a little hot sauce for a change in temperature. If shrimps are a little costly, half a pound will work just fine.

Ingredients:

1 pound shrimp, peeled, deveined and cooked
½ cup chopped onion
½ cup chopped celery
½ cup green bell pepper
1 can cream of mushroom soup
1 can cheddar cheese soup
½ cup sliced green onion
2 ¾ cups cooked rice
salt and pepper to taste
1 tablespoon butter

Directions:

Preheat oven to 350 degrees Fahrenheit. Sauté the onion, celery and bell pepper in the butter. Add the soups and heat them up. Stir in cooked rice and green onion. Remove from heat. Stir in salt and pepper. Add shrimp, mix well, and pour into a casserole dish. Bake for 20 minutes or until bubbly.

Veggie and Shrimp Ramen Noodles

Everyone knows Ramen because of its affordable price. It comes in handy in this delicious shrimp recipe.

Ingredients:

1 tablespoon toasted sesame oil
½ yellow onion, sliced
4 cups chicken stock
2 tablespoon soy sauce
1 cup asparagus pieces
1 cup bean sprouts
1 cup raw shrimp, peeled and deveined
2 Ramen packages (only noodles, not seasoning)

Directions:

Heat the sesame oil in a skillet. Sauté the onion. Pour in the chicken stock and soy sauce and mix well. Let the mixture come to a boil. Mix in the shrimp and asparagus. Cook for 3 minutes. Boil the noodles in a separate pan. Place a bed of noodles on a plate, top with bean sprouts and then with shrimp mixture to serve.

Clam Chowder

You don't have to wait until you go out to eat to have clam chowder anymore. It's easy to put together and tastes even better.

Ingredients:

2 cups chopped onion
1 ¼ cups chopped celery
½ teaspoon salt
½ teaspoon dried thyme
2 garlic cloves, minced
6 (6 ½ ounce) cans chopped clams, undrained
5 cups diced and peeled baking potatoes
4 (8 ounce) bottles clam juice
1 bay leaf
3 cups milk
½ cup all-purpose flour
2 tablespoons oil

Directions:

In a large pot, sauté the onion, celery, salt, thyme, and garlic in the oil. Drain clams and reserve liquid. Add liquid, potato, clam juice, and bay leaf to the pot and bring to a boil. Reduce heat and simmer for 15 minutes. Remove bay leaf. Whisk milk and flour together and add to the pot. Bring to a boil. Cook for 12 minutes or until thick, stirring constantly. Add clams and cook for 2 more minutes.

Tilapia with Spinach

This dinner is ready in minutes and takes away the intimidation of cooking with fresh fish. Substitute any white fish if you want.

Ingredients:

2 tilapia fillets
3 cups fresh spinach
2 cups chopped bell pepper
salt and pepper to taste
½ teaspoon garlic powder
2 teaspoons olive oil

Directions:

Heat oil up in a pan on medium-high heat. Season tilapia fillets with salt, pepper, and garlic. Place in the pan. Add spinach and bell peppers. Cover and cook, occasionally stirring the vegetables. Flip the fish halfway through. When fish is flaky and vegetables are tender, remove from pan and serve.

Garlic Shrimp Casserole

Plan ahead with this recipe when you make shrimp for dinner. This will quickly become one of your family's favorite recipes.

Ingredients:

2 cups chicken stock
2 tablespoons cornstarch mixed with 1 tablespoon water
½ cup heavy cream
½ teaspoon red pepper flakes
1 pint leftover rice
2 pints leftover garlic shrimp
¾ cup panko breadcrumbs

Directions:

Preheat oven to 350 degrees Fahrenheit. In a saucepan, combine the chicken stock and the cornstarch mixture. Simmer for 3 minutes. Add the cream and red pepper flakes. Line a terra cotta pot with foil. Pour in the rice and shrimp. Pour the cream mixture over and top with panko breadcrumbs. Bake for 45 minutes.

One-Pan Baked Salmon

Salmon is great for you but it's hard to flavor sometimes. This dish puts everything together for you and the results are amazing.

Ingredients:

4 small salmon fillets
2 cups green beans
2 cups cherry tomatoes, cut in half
2 tablespoons olive oil
2 tablespoons melted butter
1 teaspoon garlic powder
salt to taste

Directions:

Preheat oven to 400 degrees Fahrenheit. Place salmon in the middle of a baking dish. Put green beans on one side, tomatoes on the other. Drizzle vegetables with olive oil and salt, if desired. Mix the butter and garlic together and pour over salmon fillets. Bake for 20 minutes or until salmon is done.

One-Dish Italian Halibut

Who knew you could make a great dinner in the microwave? Try this halibut meal that takes the confusion out of cooking fish.

Ingredients:

2 cups instant white rice, uncooked
½ cup water
4 halibut fillets
1 (14 ½ ounce) diced tomatoes, undrained
¼ cup Italian dressing
½ cup shredded mozzarella cheese

Directions:

In a microwave safe bowl, place the rice and water in the bottom. Place fish in a single layer above. Top with tomatoes and drizzle with dressing. Cover and microwave on high for 10 minutes. Top with cheese. Microwave uncovered for 2 minutes or until fish flakes easily and rice is tender.

Chapter 5: Pork and Turkey Dinners

Pork and turkey are both typically lower in fat when compared to other meats. Try to incorporate them a few times a week.

Hungarian Pea Stew

Delicious and simple, this stew has it all. If you can't find coconut milk or sugar, regular is fine.

Ingredients:

6 cups green peas
1 pound cubed pork
2 tablespoons olive oil
3 ½ tablespoons almond flour
2 tablespoons chopped parsley
1 cup water
½ teaspoon salt
1 cup coconut milk
1 teaspoon coconut sugar

Directions:

Simmer the pork and green peas in the olive oil in a pot over medium heat for about 10 minutes. Add salt, chopped parsley, coconut sugar, and almond flour. Cook for another minute. Add water and milk. Stir well. Cook for an additional 4 minutes over low, stirring occasionally.

Sweet Pork Medallions

Just the right amount of sweet, this dish is easy with only three real ingredients. Season to taste.

Ingredients:

1 ½ pounds pork tenderloin medallions
2 tablespoons honey
4 tablespoons butter, softened
salt and pepper to taste

Directions:

Melt the butter in a skillet. Add the honey and stir. Salt and pepper each medallion and add to the skillet. Cook, about 5 minutes per side, until cooked thoroughly.

Barbecued Pork Strips

You don't need to grill to have barbecue. Serve with chips and beans.

Ingredients:

3 pounds lean pork, cut into strips
½ cup soy sauce
¼ cup dry sherry
½ cup brown sugar
2 cloves garlic, crushed
1/8 teaspoon pepper
½ cup barbecue sauce
8 ounce can pineapple chunks, undrained

Directions:

In a heavy skillet, brown pork strips in a little vegetable oil. Combine remaining ingredients in a crock-pot. Stir well. Add pork strips and stir. Cover and cook on low for 6 to 9 hours.

Baked Beans with Salt Pork

One of the most well-known combinations, this dish will please everyone. Make extra for leftovers!

Ingredients:

1 pound dried small white beans, rinsed and soaked overnight
water, to cover beans
1/3 cup molasses
¼ cup brown sugar, packed
1 cup chopped onion
¼ pound salt pork, rinsed and cut into cubes
1 tablespoon Dijon mustard
½ teaspoon salt

Directions:

Combine all ingredients, except for the salt, in a crock-pot. Cook on low 12 to 14 hours, stirring occasionally. Add salt to taste when beans are tender.

Chunky Turkey Chili

This is a healthier version of traditional chili. Go easy on the toppings for a great low calorie meal.

Ingredients:

1 pound ground turkey
½ cup chopped onion
2 (14.5 ounce) cans diced tomatoes, undrained
16 ounces pinto beans, drained and rinsed
½ cup chunky salsa
2 teaspoons chili powder
1 ½ teaspoons ground cumin
salt and pepper to taste
½ cup shredded Cheddar cheese
1 tablespoon sliced black olives

Directions:

In a large skillet, brown turkey and onion. Drain excess fat. Transfer to a crock-pot and add tomatoes, beans, salsa, chili powder, and cumin. Stir gently and cover. Cook on low for 5 to 6 hours. Season with salt and pepper. Serve with Cheddar cheese and black olives.

Turkey Breast

No more waiting until Thanksgiving for turkey. The recipe doesn't have exact amounts because you're in charge on this one. Add as little or as much as you want.

Ingredients:

1 large turkey breast
butter, as needed
potatoes, as needed
carrots, as needed
celery, as needed
onion, as needed
bell pepper, as needed
garlic powder, as needed
sage, as needed
turmeric, as needed
salt and pepper to taste

Directions:

Chop as many veggies as you would like. Rinse the turkey breast and cover with butter and seasonings. Place in a crockpot. Place vegetables around the turkey. Cover and cook for the same length as it would cook in the oven, according to package directions. When done, turn off the heat and allow to sit for 20 minutes before serving.

Apple Cider Pork

This recipe is great for a crisp fall evening. Try making it with fresh apple cider from an apple orchard.

Ingredients:

4 sweet potatoes, peeled and sliced
6 ounces dried fruit mix package
1 medium onion, sliced
1 bay leaf
¾ teaspoon salt
½ teaspoon pepper
½ teaspoon dried rosemary, crushed
1 ½ pound lean boneless pork, cut into 1 inch cubes
½ cup all-purpose flour
2 tablespoons vegetable oil
1 cup apple cider

Directions:

Heat the vegetable oil in a pan. Roll the pork in flour and season with salt and pepper. Sear in the oil on all sides. Then dump the pork and all other ingredients in a crock-pot. Cook on low for 8 to 10 hours.

Spicy Pork Chops

The perfect amount of heat is followed by the perfect amount of sweet in this pork chop meal. Serve over rice or mashed potatoes.

Ingredients:

6 boneless pork chops
½ cup honey
¼ cup cider vinegar
¼ teaspoon ground ginger
1 garlic clove, minced
2 tablespoons soy sauce
1 dash pepper

Directions:

Preheat oven to 350 degrees Fahrenheit. Place all ingredients except the pork chops in a blender. Blend together. Place the pork chops in a baking dish and pour mixture over them. Bake for 40 to 45 minutes.

Pork Chops with Rice

This dish is simple but it works great. Serve with your favorite steamed veggie.

Ingredients:

2 pork chops
salt and pepper to taste
1 clove garlic, minced
1 tablespoon brown sugar
1/8 cup soy sauce
1/6 cup chicken broth

Directions:

Place all ingredients in a crock-pot. Stir to mix well. Cover and cook on high for 5 hours. Serve over rice.

Ranch Pork Chops

Serve these pork chops over mashed potatoes for a classic dinner that will leave them wanting seconds.

Ingredients:

4 pork chops
1 packet Ranch seasoning mix
1 can cream of chicken
1 can water

Directions:

Place the pork chops in the bottom of a crock-pot. Mix other ingredients together and pour over pork chops. Cover and cook on high for 4 to 6 hours.

Sweet Pork Chops

Use any fruit preserves. Feel free to mix a couple together for your own unique combination.

Ingredients:

2 pork chops
¾ cup fruit preserves of your choice
¼ cup teriyaki sauce
1 teaspoon dried ginger
1/8 cup Dijon mustard

Directions:

Place pork chops in the bottom of a crock-pot. Mix all other ingredients together and pour over pork chops. Cover and cook on low for 6 to 8 hours.

Cheesy Pork Chops

The kids will love this one. And the best part is there's no mixing or dirtying other dishes.

Ingredients:

8 boneless pork chops, thin
1 teaspoon seasoning salt
2 cups shredded Cheddar cheese
10 teaspoons sour cream

Directions:

Preheat oven to 350 degrees Fahrenheit. Place pork chops on a baking sheet and sprinkle with seasoning salt. Cover each pork chop with sour cream and then shredded cheese. Bake for 15-20 minutes.

Creamy Pork Chops

The sauce in this recipe is beyond fabulous. Keep this recipe marked because you'll be making it again soon, guaranteed!

Ingredients:

1 package cream cheese
4 tablespoons butter
1 can cream of mushroom soup
1 package Ranch dressing mix
4-5 pork chops, frozen

Directions:

Place the frozen pork chops on the bottom of a crock-pot. Place other ingredients on top. Cook on low for 7 to 8 hours, stirring occasionally to mix ingredients.

Tuscan Pork Chops

Everything goes in one skillet and dinner appears before your eyes. Serve over a bed of pasta or zucchini noodles.

Ingredients:

4 pork chops
1 tablespoon oil
5 cloves garlic, diced
1 ½ cups fresh tomatoes, diced
1 large onion, diced
2 teaspoons oregano
1 teaspoon sage
1 teaspoon basil

Directions:

Heat oil in a large pan. Brown pork chops on each side. Reduce heat and add onions. Stir and cook for 2 minutes. Add tomatoes, garlic, and spices. Simmer until tomatoes are soft and sauce has set up.

Bleu Cheese Chops

A unique pork chop recipe, this dish only takes a few minutes to make. Whipping cream is essential for this recipe to work and cannot be substituted.

Ingredients:

2 tablespoons butter
4 pork chops
½ teaspoon pepper
½ teaspoon garlic powder
1 cup whipping cream
2 ounces bleu cheese, crumbled

Directions:

Over medium heat, melt butter. Season the pork chops with pepper and garlic. Fry in butter until no longer pink, about 20 minutes. Remove chops and keep warm on a plate. Stir the whipping cream into the skillet, then bleu cheese. Stir constantly for 5 minutes or until sauce thickens. Pour over pork chops.

Turkey Casserole

This casserole is perfect for company. Double or triple it for large groups or parties.

Ingredients:

2 onions, chopped
1 green pepper, chopped
2 tablespoons butter
6 cups cubed cooked turkey
2 cans cream of chicken soup
2 cups sour cream
1 package frozen chopped spinach, thawed and squeezed dry
2 cups shredded Monterey Jack cheese
1 package tortilla chips, crushed

Directions:

Preheat oven to 350 degrees Fahrenheit. Grease a 9 x 13 inch baking pan. Sauté onions and green pepper in butter in a pot. Stir in turkey, soup, sour cream, and spinach. Place half in the baking pan. Add a layer of cheese and a layer of chips. Repeat layers. Bake for 25 to 30 minutes or until bubbly.

Turkey and Broccoli Casserole

If you have leftover turkey, this is how you should use it. Chicken can be substituted as well.

Ingredients:

¼ cup chopped onion
¼ cup chopped celery
¼ cup butter, cubed
4 cups cubed turkey breast, cooked
1 package frozen broccoli, thawed
1 can cream of mushroom soup
1 can cream of chicken soup
1 cup rice, cooked
½ cup shredded mozzarella cheese
1 can French-fried onions

Directions:

Preheat oven to 350 degrees Fahrenheit. Sauté onion and celery in butter. Stir in the turkey, broccoli, soups and rice. Transfer to a baking dish. Bake for 25-30 minutes or until bubbly Sprinkle with cheese and French-fried onions and bake for 5 more minutes.

Chapter 6: Vegetarian Dinners and Sides

Here are some great vegetarian and side dish options to either add to another dump dinner or serve alone. Many will work great as a lunch option as well.

Crock-Pot Eggplant

Garnish with fresh basil leaves and leaf lettuce if desired.

Ingredients:

1 ¼ pounds eggplant, cut into 1 inch cubes
2 onions, sliced
2 ribs celery, cut into 1 inch pieces
1 tablespoon olive oil
1 (16 ounce) can diced tomatoes, undrained
3 tablespoons tomato sauce
½ cup pitted ripe olives, cut in half
2 tablespoons balsamic vinegar
1 tablespoon sugar
1 tablespoon capers, drained
1 teaspoon dried oregano
salt and pepper to taste

Directions:

Place the eggplant, onion, celery, tomatoes, tomato sauce, and oil in a crock-pot. Cover and cook for 4 hours on low or until the eggplant is tender. Mix in the olives, sugar, capers, vinegar, and oregano. Cook for 1 more hour. Add salt and pepper to taste and serve with any desired garnish.

Brown Potato Soup

Potato soup is a classic and this recipe is sure to become a favorite. Change the type of cheese if you would like.

Ingredients:

32 ounces frozen Southern-style diced hash browns
½ cup frozen chopped onion
½ cup diced celery
32 ounces chicken broth
1 cup water
3 tablespoons flour
2 cups shredded Cheddar cheese
1 cup milk

Directions:

Place all ingredients in a crock-pot. Cook on low for 6-8 hours.

Mexican Dip

This can work as an appetizer or a main course. Serve over rice or just with the chips.

Ingredients:

1 (10 ounce) package frozen chopped spinach, thawed and drained
1 (8 ounce) package shredded Mexican blend cheese
1 package cream cheese, at room temperature
1 cup half and half
1 (15 ounce) jar medium salsa
1 teaspoon chili powder
tortilla chips, for serving

Directions:

Preheat oven to 350 degrees Fahrenheit. Mix all of the ingredients except for the chips in a large bowl, making sure that there are no lumps. Transfer to a baking dish. Bake for 30 minutes or until cheese is melted.

Barbecue Bean Soup

Perfect for a lazy night, this recipe makes plenty and freezes well.

Ingredients:

1 pound navy beans, soaked overnight and simmered until tender
¾ cup chopped onion
1 teaspoon salt
1/8 teaspoon pepper
6 cups water
¾ cup barbecue sauce

Directions:

Drain cooked beans. Combine all ingredients in a crock-pot. Cover and cook on low for 7 to 9 hours.

Baked Pineapple Stuffing

A fun twist on a classic, the pineapple gives this stuffing a tropical flavor.

Ingredients:

20-ounce can crushed pineapple, undrained
¼ cup evaporated milk
1 cup packaged cornbread stuffing crumbs
¾ cup sugar
¼ cup melted butter
3 eggs, beaten

Directions:

Lightly grease the bottom and sides of a crock-pot. Combine all ingredients in the crock-pot. Cover and cook on high for 2 to 3 hours.

Cheesy Hash Browns

This recipe is great for dinner or breakfast. Everyone will love these hash browns.

Ingredients:

1 bag frozen hash browns
8 ounces sour cream
1 can cream of chicken soup
¼ cup diced onion
1 ½ cups shredded Cheddar cheese
½ cup butter, melted
salt and pepper to taste

Directions:

Mix the hash browns, sour cream, soup, onion, cheese, and melted butter in a bowl. Dump into a crock-pot. Sprinkle with salt and pepper and cover. Cook on low for 4 to 5 hours.

Ginger Potato Casserole

This is a perfect side dish for a fancy meal. If you can't find ginger garlic paste, it's easy to make your own.

Ingredients:

2 tablespoons ginger garlic paste
2 potatoes, boiled
1 bunch spring onion, chopped
1 cup cheese
1 green pepper, chopped
2 small carrots, chopped
2 tablespoons oil
salt and pepper to taste

Directions:

Preheat oven to 350 degrees Fahrenheit. Spray a baking dish. Add all of the ingredients except for the cheese to the dish and mix well. Bake until bubbly, about 20 minutes. Top with cheese and bake for 5 more minutes.

Mushroom Macaroni

Who said macaroni can't be healthy? Fresh or canned mushrooms work in this recipe.

Ingredients:

1 box of macaroni, prepared
¼ cup mushrooms
1 teaspoon olive oil
salt and pepper to taste
1 cup cheese
½ cup milk
½ cup cream

Directions:

Preheat oven to 350 degrees Fahrenheit. Mix all ingredients except for the cheese together. Pour into a baking dish and top with cheese. Bake for 20-30 minutes.

Tofu Fajitas

If you're never tried tofu, this is how you should experience it. Serve with tortillas or over rice.

Ingredients:

2 teaspoons chili powder
1 pound tofu
2 teaspoons cumin
2 tablespoons vegetable oil
½ teaspoon dried oregano
1 teaspoon garlic powder
1 can diced tomatoes
1 onion, sliced
2 green bell peppers, sliced
flour tortillas

Directions:

Preheat oven to 400 degrees Fahrenheit. Place the tofu in a 9 x 13 baking dish. Mix together the oil, chili powder, cumin, salt, oregano, and garlic powder in a bowl. Spread over the tofu, coating both sides. Add the onions, peppers and tomatoes, stirring well. Bake for 10-15 minutes or until vegetables are tender.

Red Beans and Rice

This is great as a simple side dish or a full meal. Mix up the types of rice and beans to your personal taste.

Ingredients:

2 cups brown rice
3 cloves garlic, minced
1 can dark red kidney beans
2 teaspoons paprika
4 cups vegetable stock
salt and pepper to taste

Directions:

Add all ingredients to a large pot. Cover and simmer until all of the liquid is absorbed. Limit opening the lid so that steam doesn't escape.

Spinach Ravioli Bake

This meal is filling and delicious. Add other vegetables if desired.

Ingredients:

2 cans spaghetti sauce
1 pack frozen, chopped spinach
1 bag frozen ravioli
2 cups shredded mozzarella cheese
¼ cup grated Parmesan cheese

Directions:

Preheat oven to 350 degrees Fahrenheit. Thaw the spinach and squeeze all the excess water out. Spread one cup of spaghetti sauce on the bottom of a 9 x 13 baking dish. Top it with half the bag of ravioli, half of the mozzarella, and half of the Parmesan. Repeat this process. Bake for 40 to 45 minutes, until cheese is melted.

Garlic and Cheese Potatoes

The name says it all. This recipe is the perfect combination of all things delicious.

Ingredients:

1/3 cup melted butter
1/3 cup breadcrumbs
1 ½ pounds unpeeled red potatoes, cut in half
1 cup Cheddar cheese
2 cloves garlic
½ teaspoon paprika
salt and pepper to taste

Directions:

Preheat oven to 375 degrees Fahrenheit. In a bowl, mix butter and garlic. Add potatoes and toss to coat. Add the rest of the ingredients and stir well. Spread the coated potatoes on a baking sheet. Bake for one hour, flipping a few times throughout.

Coconut Rice

Try this sweetened rice that's almost considered a dessert.

Ingredients:

1 ½ cups dry Jasmine rice
1 (15 ounce) coconut milk
2 cloves garlic
1 cup water
salt to taste

Directions:

Rinse the rice until water is no longer cloudy. Add all ingredients to a pot and stir. Cook over high heat until the mixture comes to a boil. Turn down heat and simmer for 30 minutes, covered. Remove from heat and let sit for 15 minutes.

Cheesy Bread Rolls

These bread rolls will go fast. Try dipped in ranch or melted herb butter.

Ingredients:

1 tube (10 pieces) flaky dinner rolls
2 tablespoons butter, melted
½ cup shredded Cheddar cheese
2 tablespoons mozzarella cheese
1 teaspoon dried parsley
1 teaspoon dried oregano
½ teaspoon garlic powder
salt to taste

Directions:

Preheat oven to 375 degrees Fahrenheit. Cut each roll into four pieces. Dump all ingredients in a bowl and stir to coat the bread pieces. Pour into a 9 x 13 baking dish and bake for 12 to 15 minutes or until bread is golden brown.

Lemon and Herb Orzo

The lemon adds a great kick to the orzo in this recipe. Try to use fresh herbs for a real flavor boost.

Ingredients:

1 ½ cups orzo
4 cups water
3 tablespoons butter
1 cup chopped parsley
1 cup chives
1 cup chopped dill
zest of 1 lemon
salt and pepper to taste

Directions:

Cook orzo in salted boiling water. Drain, reserving ¼ cup of cooking water. Toss orzo with butter, salt, pepper, dill, chives, parsley, and lemon zest. Mix in the reserved cooking water, if more moisture is needed.

Lentil Soup

Lentil soup is a favorite of many and this recipe won't disappoint. The beans don't have to be soaked beforehand so it's quick to come together too.

Ingredients:

2 cups dried red lentils
32 ounces vegetable broth
3 carrots, cut into chunks
1 can diced tomatoes
4 ounces tomato paste
1 onion, diced
2 garlic cloves, minced
1 teaspoon dried basil
1 teaspoon dried them
½ teaspoon ground cumin
1 teaspoon salt
¼ teaspoon pepper

Directions:

Place all ingredients in a crock-pot. Cover and cook on low for 8 to 10 hours or on high for 4 to 5 hours, stirring occasionally.

Cheese Pizza

Stop ordering pizza and make your own with this easy version. Add other toppings as desired.

Ingredients:

1 (13 ounce) refrigerated pizza crust
1 ½ cups pizza sauce
2 ½ cups of pizza cheese mix
1/3 cup Parmesan cheese

Directions:

Preheat oven to 425 degrees Fahrenheit. Grease a 9 x 13 baking pan. Unroll the pizza dough and press into the bottom of the pan and also halfway up each side. Spread with pizza sauce and top with cheese. Bake for 15 to 20 minutes or until crust is golden brown and cheese is melted.

Cheese Tortellini

This recipe is creamy and rich. You won't believe the taste after seeing how fast it comes together.

Ingredients:

1 bag cheese tortellini, frozen
1 small bag of fresh spinach
2 (14.5 ounce) cans of Italian style diced tomatoes, drained
1 package cream cheese
3 cups vegetable broth

Directions:

Place all ingredients in a crock-pot. Stir well. Cover and cook on low for 4 to 6 hours.

Veggie Casserole

Use up all the leftover frozen veggies in the freezer with this casserole. Works as a main dish or a quick side dish.

Ingredients:

2 tablespoons butter
½ onion, diced
1 carrot, diced
½ cup corn
2 cups broccoli florets
1 can cream of celery soup
salt and pepper to taste
2 pinches ground thyme
1 cup long grain white rice
2 cups water
1 ½ cups shredded Cheddar cheese

Directions:

Preheat oven to 350 degrees Fahrenheit. Sauté onions, carrot, and corn in butter. Stir in broccoli and soup. Add seasonings, rice, and water. Mix well while the mixture heats. Melt cheese in and then pour into a baking dish. Bake for 40 minutes or until rice is cooked.

Chapter 7: Bonus Desserts

Now don't think that we would only give you dinner recipes. Life's too short not to have dessert! Here's a few bonus dessert recipes that you can whip together in a flash, perfect for special occasions or just because.

Chocolate Pudding Cake

Chocolate, pudding, and cake is perfection. Serve warm with ice cream.

Ingredients:

1 box chocolate cake mix
1 small instant chocolate pudding mix
1 ½ cups milk
1 ½ cups chocolate chips

Directions:

Preheat oven to 350 degrees Fahrenheit. Combine the dry cake mix, dry pudding mix, and milk in a bowl. Mix well. Spread into a greased 9 x 13 baking dish. Top with the

RUTH FERGUSON

chocolate chips. Bake for about 30 minutes or until the edges begin to pull away from the pan.

Apple Dump Cake

This cake comes together in minutes and fills the house with a fabulous scent. Add a sprinkle of cinnamon sugar before serving.

Ingredients:

1 dry box yellow cake mix (with ingredients needed for cake)
2 (21 ounce) cans apple pie mix
1 stick butter
½ cup water

Directions:

Preheat oven to 350 degrees Fahrenheit. Spray a 9 x 13 inch cake pan. Place the apple pie mix on the bottom. Mix the cake mix according to the box directions. Pour on top of the apples. Melt the butter with the water and pour on top of the cake batter. Bake for 70 minutes.

Cherry Dump Cake

This recipe has a few more ingredients than most dump cakes but you will be rewarded.

Ingredients:

1 can (21 ounces) cherry pie filling
2 cups all-purpose flour
2 teaspoons baking powder
1 ¼ cup sugar
2 eggs
½ cup butter, softened
½ teaspoon salt
1 teaspoon grated lemon zest
1 teaspoon vanilla extract

Directions:

Preheat oven to 350 degrees Fahrenheit. Grease and flour a 9 x 13 cake pan. Dump the cherry pie filling in. Mix the flour, baking powder, sugar, eggs, butter, salt, lemon zest, and vanilla together in a bowl. Dump over the cherry filling. Bake for 1 hour.

Banana Split Dump Cake

If you can't make the sundae, this cake will settle your craving. Serve with sliced bananas, whipped cream, and chocolate sauce.

Ingredients:

1 (21 ounce) can strawberry pie filling
1 (20 ounce) can crushed pineapple, undrained
1 white cake mix
1 stick margarine, cut in pieces
1 cup coconut
½ tablespoon crushed nuts

Directions:

Preheat the oven to 325 degrees Fahrenheit. Grease a 9 x 13 cake pan. Spread the strawberry filling on the bottom. Spread the pineapple on top and then the dry cake mix. Sprinkle the margarine pieces over the cake mix. Top with coconut and crushed nuts. Bake for 60-75 minutes. Top with desired toppings.

Pumpkin Dump Cake

Perfect in the fall or any time of year, this cake will earn you great reviews. Make sure to use only pumpkin and not pumpkin pie mix.

Ingredients:

1 large can pumpkin
1 can (12 ounces) nonfat evaporated milk
4 eggs
1 cup white sugar
1 teaspoon ground nutmeg
1 teaspoon ground ginger
1 teaspoon ground cloves
2 teaspoons ground cinnamon
½ teaspoon salt
1 package yellow cake mix
½ cup butter, melted
1 cup chopped pecans

Directions:

Preheat oven to 350 degrees Fahrenheit. Grease and flour a 9 x 13 cake pan. Mix the pumpkin, sugar, salt, nutmeg, ginger, cloves, and cinnamon together in a large bowl. Stir in the milk and then the eggs, one at a time. Pour the mixture into the pan. Pour the cake mix over the pumpkin and then top with pecans. Drizzle melted butter over all. Bake for 45-55 minutes.

A Little Food For Thought...

So many people turn to expensive and unhealthy take-out meals these days because they just don't think that they have the time to put a home-cooked meal on the table for their family. The nights that they do spend cooking leave them drained and discouraged when they see that they spent more time making the meal than it took their family to eat. After cleaning up, the night is over and they are left wondering what the point of it was.

But with dump dinners, you get the best of both worlds. Your family will get a home-cooked meal that won't break the bank while you still get time to relax and enjoy your evening at home. It's easier than you think and should leave you with more money, more time and less stress. Chances are that you have everything you need in your kitchen right now to make your first dump dinner tonight! Won't your family be pleasantly surprised to see you relaxing while a dump dinner virtually cooks itself?

I urge you to give the world of dump dinners a try. Your first recipe might not go perfectly but that's okay. Every type of cooking has a bit of a learning curve. Before you know it, you'll be making dinner every night in only minutes while your friends ask what your secret is. You can rest assured that your family will appreciate you giving dump dinners a try, especially once these delicious meals are flying out of your kitchen every night.

Enjoy!

Ruthie

www.ingramcontent.com/pod-product-compliance
Lightning Source LLC
Chambersburg PA
CBHW021446070526
44577CB00002B/286